THIS BOOK IS PRIVATE

So don't read it. If found please return it to:

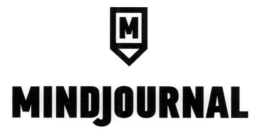

MINDJOURNAL

This book will make you stronger

EBURY
PRESS

CONTENTS

INTRODUCTION

08
HEY MAN. WHAT'S UP!?

10
WELCOME TO THE MOVEMENT

14
WHAT IS JOURNALING?

20
WHY I KEEP A JOURNAL

26
HOW MINDJOURNAL WORKS

28
THE WRITING PROGRAMME

THE JOURNAL

34
STAGE ONE — WARM UP

78
STAGE TWO — HURDLES

122
STAGE THREE — STRENGTH

SUPPORT GUIDE

170
PERMISSIONS

172
CHECK YO' SELF

174
STRESS TEST

176
NEGOTIATING

178
RECHARGE

180
PERFORMANCE

182
FAQs

186
LIFELINES

188
LOOK AFTER YOURSELF

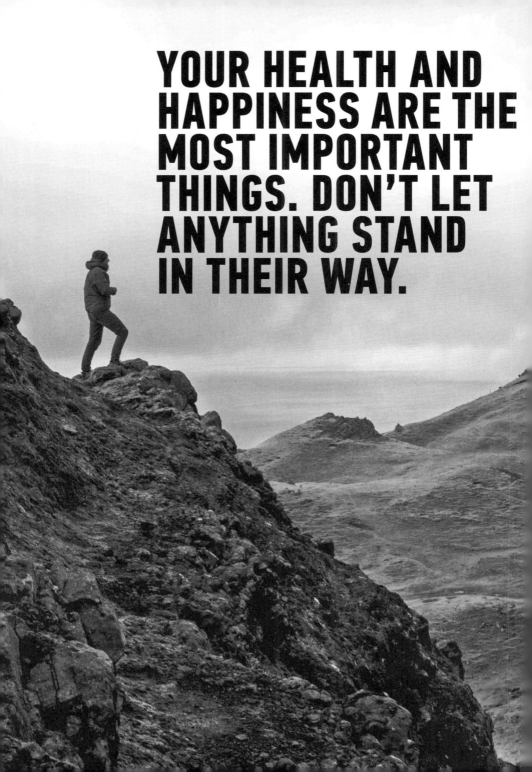

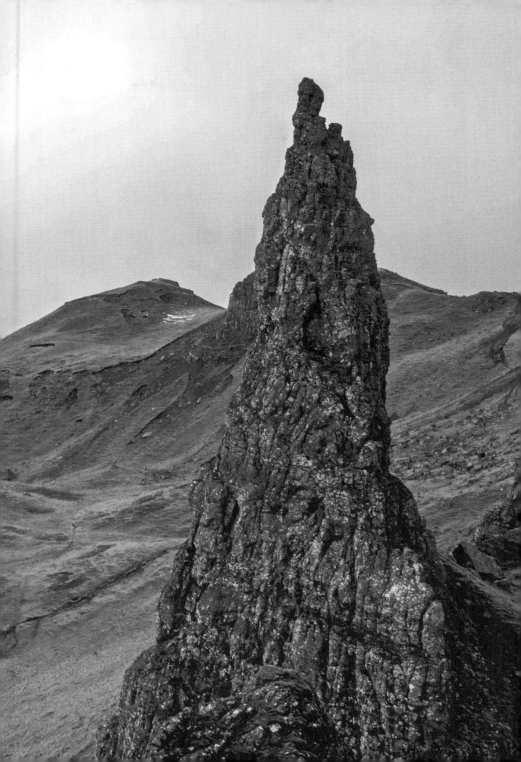

HEY MAN.
WHAT'S UP!?

There's a reason you're here. And I don't know what that is. But over the coming days, weeks, months or even years, you and this book are going to get to know each other pretty damn well.

You don't have to have a problem to be reading this. I don't want to talk to you like a doctor or a therapist. I'm just going to talk to you like a mate. From one ordinary guy to another. It will never be any more complicated than that.

The aim of this book is to help and support you through life's daily ups and downs. The good, the bad and all the stuff in between. It really doesn't matter what's going on in your life just use this as a safe place to vent everything that is. This is about you having a new tool to use that will help you be a stronger version of the man you already are.

Life is constantly throwing up challenges. And often we find ourselves battling through. I know because I've been there and still find life hardwork. What I've learned along the way, though, is that life is for the making. And that when your mind is in the right place, you cope better, feel happier and achieve a whole lot more.

I'm beyond grateful that you're here — I promise that you won't regret it. Just before you dive in, though, I want to remind you to look after yourself during this journey. Enjoy it. Have fun. And thanks again for being here.

Ollie Aplin
Founder of MindJournal

WELCOME TO THE MOVEMENT

Damn right this is a movement. And it's just getting started. There literally could not be a better time than now to get into journaling.

And how did this all start? Well, the idea for this book came from a chat I was having with a friend, in a pub, over a beer. He mentioned he was having a rough time of things and I suggested he keep a journal. Solid advice it seemed. Until he came back to me and said he'd given it a try but couldn't get into it. When I asked why, he just said he didn't know where to start. And that got me thinking.

When I first started keeping a journal years ago, I battled with it. It felt completely unnatural. Writing down everything you think and feel. In a book. I couldn't get into it either. But my therapist at the time advised I stick to it. And with her support, I managed to build up the confidence and skill required to journal freely.

So I completely related with the struggle my friend had found with his journal. And after a bit of digging around the internet, I found tons of other people struggling with the concept of journaling. It was at this point I realised what I needed to do. Make a journal that actually helps you keep one.

Not long after I started designing it though I realised that most of my circle of friends, colleagues and connections were guys. And I find chatting to blokes about stuff a lot more comfortable than I do women. This is when I had my second light-bulb moment — to make the journal exclusively for us chaps. MindJournal officially launched on Kickstarter, a hugely popular crowd-funding platform, back in February 2016. And after just 72 hours the campaign smashed through its original funding goal.

By June 2016 we shipped out hundreds of journals to guys all across the world From North and South America to Australia and New Zealand. Even to guys out in Asia and the Middle East.

I had self-published an international journal and I was absolutely speechless at what had been achieved.

I was moved and overwhelmed to say the least. Not by the figures but by the stories from guys that showed their support for the campaign. The Kickstarter inspired an army of men to take action on how to deal with everyday life. And help reassure those same guys that, no matter what they were experiencing, there was now a tool to help them find their inner strength.

And this is the movement. Guys back doing what guys do well — journaling. You are now part of the movement. A huge, global mission that aims to bring back the power of journaling.

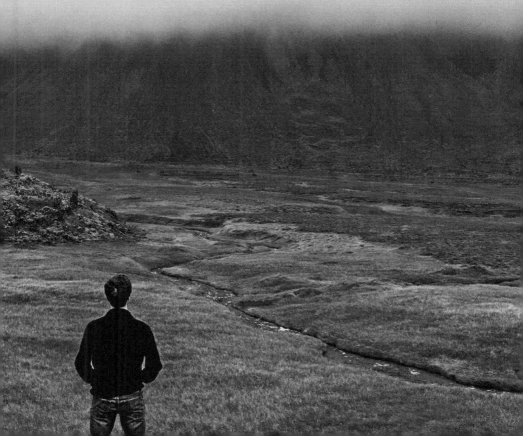

USING MINDJOURNAL HAS HAD A HUGE IMPACT ON MY LIFE. WHENEVER I FEEL ALONE, CONFUSED OR HAPPY, I NOW WRITE MY THOUGHTS DOWN.

ALEXANDER, 32 — MINDJOURNAL USER, GERMANY

WHAT IS JOURNALING?

You don't have to be nuts or have problems to keep a journal. It's a healthy habit that everyone could be doing more of.

It's a solid, robust life tool that will help you feel stronger and better equipped to handle whatever life throws you. No matter your past, present or future.

First off, journaling is not the same as keeping a diary. Writing a journal sounds way cooler but it's also a lot more personal than a diary. Diaries tend to be used to record specific daily activities and are usually written in chronological order. Journaling is more about experiences, thoughts and emotions. And there is no expectation to write daily, just when you feel the need.

Back in the day, keeping a journal was a manly thing to do. All the great thinkers, writers and explorers of the past kept a journal on a regular basis from Ernest Hemingway to Kurt Cobain and Bruce Lee. It was a simple habitual practice. A pipe, a drink and a break in the day to write everything that was on your mind. Writing as a therapeutic outlet, particularly for men, has sadly been lost over time. I want to bring it back. Minus the pipe and booze. But with that original sense of pride for keeping a journal. Something you look forward to doing. Something that becomes part of your life. Part of your style. And part of who you are.

I know the importance and power of journaling and I want it to become seamless in the lives of men. Journaling should be an activity that we enjoy. It should speak to us in the same language we use in our day-to-day lives. I want journaling to feel as natural as visiting the barbers, hitting the gym or any of the other things us guys do ordinarily.

Take skincare for example. My face would look proper ropey if I didn't do my morning moisturise routine. I couldn't have said that a few years back. But look at us now 'manscaping' away: barbers, gym, post-gym shakes and even skincare — all in an effort to feel good about ourselves. Does it work? Or is it just a way to put more stress, pressure and expectations on ourselves? To look a certain way. To perform at an increasing capacity.

This is where the power of journaling cuts through the bullshit. Because it's you talking to you. No one is telling you what to say, how to feel or what to do. You make the rules, you define your own journey. I don't want you to keep a journal because I'm telling you to. I want you to want to keep a journal for you.

The job of this book is to prove to you that journaling can help, whatever the situation you find yourself in. No matter how busy you are or how bad your handwriting is. Just the motion of moving the pen around the page helps to unlock those trapped thoughts and feelings within you. When the pen is moving, it's like the stuff in your brain is literally pouring out of your head, down your arm, through your hand, into the pen, out of the ink and on to the page.

Keeping a journal gives you back control over your thoughts and allows you to carve out time just for you. This is the most crucial thing to remember. And if you're a bit of a sceptic, like my old man, there's tons of science out there to support the fact that journaling is packed full of benefits.

Early on in the inception of MindJournal I spoke to Karen Pine, a friend of mine who is a psychology professor in all this stuff. She helped me understand the more scientific side to journaling via the work of Professor James Pennebaker. His studies showed that people who were asked to write down their deepest thoughts and feelings were able to handle past traumas and emotional stress significantly better than those who didn't write anything down.

Crucially, he found that it didn't matter what words were written but it was more the act of expressing the feelings by getting them down on paper.

On top of that, Professor Pennebaker's research has shown that for people who are not comfortable talking to a stranger, for fear of being judged, writing offers a less stressful alternative to seeing a therapist. Especially for men who have been brought up to hide their feelings or come from families where emotions weren't discussed. Like myself.

I was raised not to speak of the things going on at home. My journal was the first place I had to put all the thoughts that I wasn't allowed to share with anyone else. And I didn't have to worry about sounding weak or upsetting others.

If the thought of keeping a journal fills you with dread, bear with me. I can promise you that when you're done, the feeling of relief will massively outweigh the anxiety you had before. That jumbled mess of noise, feelings, words and memories will finally be quiet. You'll feel calmer and clearer.

You already have all the answers to the toughest questions that you're too afraid to ask. This book will teach you to face those questions, and begin the journey to finding your own answers.

A JOURNAL IS LIKE
A LETTERBOX. IF YOU
ONLY POST BULLSHIT,
THEN THAT'S ALL
YOU'LL EVER READ.

BE HONEST.
BE TRUE.
BE YOU.

WHY I KEEP A JOURNAL

You're probably wondering 'who the hell is this guy!?'.

Born to a bipolar mum, life was never going to be straightforward. My parents split when I was around 4 years old. My sister and I lived with mum. Dad remarried and moved abroad and, when I was 13, my sister left home so it was just me and mum.

From the drinking and suicide attempts to the pure love and protection she gave, life with mum was a volatile mix of extreme highs and lows. The hardest thing in the world is to watch someone you love the most, try and destroy themselves while you're helpless to save them. That was my relationship with mum during most of my teenage years. And my way of coping was drink, drugs and, oddly, design.

My close circle of friends all had their own shit going on and we bonded through drinking and drug taking. The streets became a second home. I stayed out all hours, dodging other fucked-up kids that wanted to rob or fight us.

By the time I turned 17, home life was more extreme. In mum's mind, she believed that by ending her life I would be set free. A few months after booting me out of the house, after a row we had, she succeeded in calling it a day for good. On Tuesday 22nd November 2005 the police informed me, on the steps of what once was home, that my mum was dead. All the events that followed are either a blur or burnt into my memory like a hot iron. One of which was identifying her body in the hospital morgue and begging her to wake up.

Afterwards I was plagued with anxiety, panic attacks, post-traumatic stress and crippling headaches. Somehow I had survived everything and also held it together. Then, almost two Years after her death, I suffered a mental breakdown.

I questioned my own sanity. Did all of that actually happen? Where is mum now? What the fuck is going on and why can't I stop crying? I just wanted to sleep but couldn't. I was starving but didn't want to eat. I couldn't work, socialise or function as a human being.

Eventually, and after some help, I realised I wasn't alone in what I was experiencing. I had survived my mum's suicide. And there were other survivors out there. What I was experiencing was normal. As un-normal as it actually felt. Funnily enough I was probably the sanest I'd ever been.

I started therapy. Started journaling. And started living.

To get to where I am now has taken me eleven years. I still have anxiety, panic attacks and these damn headaches but I've learned to live with them. I've learned to carry on living. And I've discovered a number of tools along the way that help keep me on track. And they are writing, talking and exercising. If I stop doing any one of these things, everything goes sideways pretty damn quick.

I've been keeping a journal since 2008 and it's not something I've ever found easy. The idea of pouring out my lows and highs on to blank paper is a daunting one. Even if I do know the benefits, staring at that crisp whiteness, that void of emptiness, just swallows me up.

When I was advised to keep a journal by my therapist, I found it almost impossible. At that time in my life I had feelings that I didn't understand. Feelings I couldn't connect with and didn't really want to feel, let alone talk or write about.

I'm someone that's been raised to suppress their feelings in order to protect those around me. Bit by bit I got there. It took time, patience and support and I grew stronger and stronger.

That's my story, yours might be similar or completely different. And I just want to be clear: this journal is not about me. It's about you and your journey. You can and will do all of it by yourself.

I'm only here to share with you all the tools I've learned, that have helped give me the strength to survive all the things I've been through. I will say, though, that the biggest lesson I've learned through my entire life is to not be afraid to ask for help. Don't ever be afraid to stick your hand up.

I can't promise you that this book will solve all your issues. I don't have all the answers. I am not a life guru. In fact I'm still finding things out myself. I'm just a normal guy that's been through some stuff and knows what it's like when the seas go from rough to calm and back to rough again. You're not alone. And never will be. And that's all you need to remember.

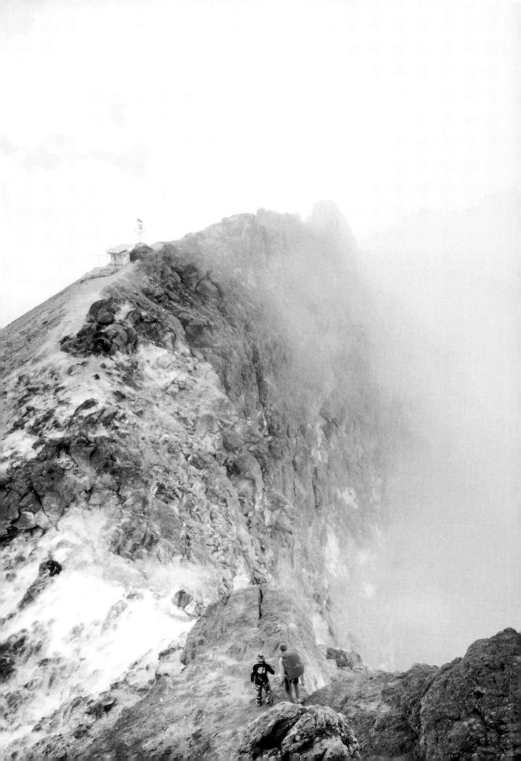

NOTHING WORTH DOING IS EVER EASY.

GREAT THINGS HAPPEN WHEN YOU STEP OUTSIDE YOUR COMFORT ZONE.

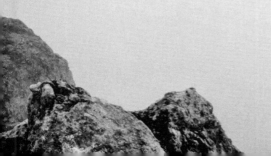

HOW MINDJOURNAL WORKS

MindJournal's strength lies in its simplicity. What's been created is a Writing Programme that actively gets you writing.

The main reason people don't keep a journal is that they don't know where to start when they come to write in one. And I know exactly what this feels like. When your mind is filled to the brim with stuff, it's hard to find focus let alone the words to write.

But using this journal will help you find that focus and those words. How? By giving you a series of highly constructed questions and prompts called Thought Triggers that will help kick things off for you, whenever you come to write. Cos' that's the hardest bit: getting started.

This unique journal will encourage you to be you. Connecting with yourself is true strength. Strength you can't build down the gym.

A shed load of research and man-hours of speaking with therapists and psychologists along the way have led to this book. It hasn't just been cobbled together by some anxiety-suffering nut-case. It's been tested, and then tested some more. And thanks to feedback from all the guys using the Kickstarter edition, I've been able to create the ultimate Writing Programme.

This new book is a completely reworked product, filled to the brim with new prompts and tasks — it's guaranteed to leave your mind blown. The power behind each prompt is now revealed, and I've written a detailed breakdown of each and every Thought Trigger in the Writing Programme.

By the time you get to the end of this book, you'll have completed your first journal. Not only this you'll be in a more positive and stronger position to tackle journaling. And whatever life throws at you next.

THE WRITING PROGRAMME

The core journal part of this book has been designed to feel doable. Something that doesn't feel like a mission or a chore. And to achieve this, the journal has been broken down into three core stages— Warm Up, Hurdles and Strength.

Within each of these stages comes a set of ten exercises for you to work through. Each exercise is formed of four key components, Thought Triggers, Feelings, Support from me and a Lined Area for you to write your entry.

This then repeats. By repeating this process you'll build up your writing so it becomes habitual. Over time you will start to ask your own questions and you'll have the confidence and know-how to kick-off your own writing sessions.

The programme also gets more engaging the more you use it. With powerful chunks of inspiration and challenging tasks, the journal will keep you on your toes — tackling all the ways we learn.

Yes you are writing but this journal will help you to engage with things around you in a different way. It's a journey of you discovering more about you as you go.

1 WARM UP

The mind is like a muscle and it needs warming up before you get it working. This first section is like a bit of light stretching for the brain. Starting off with simple Thought Triggers that will vary from drawing charts to writing raps. All nice and easy to help you loosen those fingers and get your mind all warmed up. This section gets you thinking about the past and how your life is now.

2 HURDLES

By now you should be nicely warmed up and have a good idea of what's going on. Now let's get the heart pumping. The second batch of Thought Triggers are tougher so be prepared to push yourself. This section is all about you and the people around you. It will highlight your strengths and weaknesses. It's only after you've recognised your limitations and barriers that you can then figure out how to get over them.

3 STRENGTH

Time to step things up and load up the rack. This is where you'll become a pro journaler. The Thought Triggers here will push, pull and test your endurance. But you've proved you can do it. Nothing worth doing is ever easy. And you're going to be blown away with what you can achieve when you put your mind to it. This last section gets you thinking about your needs and your future, so you can live life stronger.

BASIC INSTRUCTIONS

As the late Tupac Shakur once wrote, 'it's all about you'. There are no rules to keeping a journal. No right or wrong way of doing this.

Just do whatever feels right for you. Here are some pointers, though, that might help you on your way:

1. Always try answering the Thought Trigger first

2. Then highlight how you're feeling

3. Try to use your journal at least once a week

4. Allocate 15-30 minutes for each session

5. Write somewhere quiet with no distractions

6. Always date your entries to check your progress

7. Writing one word or sentence is OK

8. Don't worry about your spelling or handwriting

9. Keep it somewhere safe

10. Make it a habit, create a routine

11. Be honest and let loose

12. Enjoy the journey

SUPPORT GUIDE

At the back of this journal you'll find an additional support area to help you if you get stuck or feel a bit crap.

This writing journey is not supposed to be easy. Nothing worth doing ever is. I found that keeping a journal opened up a voice inside me that had lain dormant my entire life. It opened up my mind and shed light on things that I'd never given much thought to before. Particularly, on how to really look after myself, something which I'm still learning about.

The support guide at the back of the book will help you with all the core areas of mind-maintenance. From stress to rest, it's got you covered. Here's a breakdown of what you'll find:

page 170 — **Permissions**

page 172 — **Check Yo' Self**

page 1174 — **Stress Test**

page 176 — **Negotiating**

page 178 — **Recharge**

page 180 — **Performance**

page 182 — **FAQs**

page 186 — **Lifelines**

YOU'RE ABOUT TO
EMBARK ON AN
INCREDIBLE JOURNEY.

AND EVEN THOUGH THE
TERRAIN MIGHT GET
ROCKY AND ROUGH,
THE VIEW AT THE END
WILL BE WORTH IT.

BE BRAVE.
YOU CAN DO THIS.

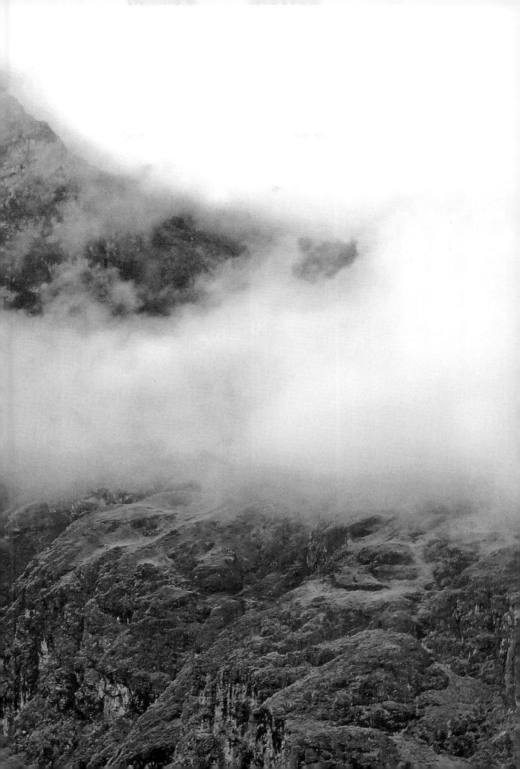

STAGE ONE
WARM UP

1

This is the first stage you're going to work through. Over the next few pages you'll find the first ten Thought Triggers to help get things going.

Like all exercises, it's good to do some stretches first. Warm up those muscles. Get in the zone.

You might find your mind wandering while thinking about the Thought Trigger that you've just read. This stage is about learning to capture those thoughts and feelings and put them down on paper. Giving them a place to live that's not just in your head, cluttering up all the other stuff you've got going on up there.

Knowing why you are being asked to do something is important too. By knowing the why, it will help you with the what. So an overview of each Thought Trigger has been provided to help you even more. Learning new things helps us grow as individuals. And this journey is about more than just learning a new skill, you're learning how to use a new tool.

Welcome to the first session man. Now let's get going.

ENTRY ONE
YOUR GOALS

The amazing thing about goals is that they're
more about the journey, rather than
the destination.

I've continuously set myself goals over the years. Some I've reached. Some I've failed. And some I later realised weren't really goals at all.

What I've found is that the journey is way more important than the destination. It's not about the outcome, but the steps along the way that help us build strength.

There's a bucket load of data, research and studies into the value of goal setting. And there's a knack to getting it right. So before you plough into the first task, have a think. Be honest with yourself. And allow yourself the time to really stretch your brain and think about what specific goals you'd like to explore. I'd aim for around two or three. Don't over do it and put too much pressure on yourself. Try to think outside your comfort zone. Your goals should be tough but not impossible. Think about the words you use. Give your goals a positive vibe, it will help you focus on what you want in your life.

The main thing to remember is that your goals shouldn't be overly complex. They should be fun and exciting. So when you're ready, think, feel and then write them down.

WHAT ARE YOUR GOALS?

Why did you decide to embark on this journey? What would
you like to get from doing this? Is there a bigger goal
that you're aiming for?

HOW ARE YOU FEELING?

Circle, tick or cross out

stressed nervous tense anxious insecure confused
positive happy hopeful determined glad joyful proud
bored tired hurt angry irritated disappointed annoyed
motivated eager excited content daring safe inspired
frustrated furious scared trapped worthless unhappy
calm grateful strong neutral empathetic mischievous alive
regretful upset lonely low guilty bitter shocked sad
confident pleased surprised relieved satisfied energetic

If the idea of writing is still freaking you out, give
yourself the permission to do this. Head to page
170 in the Support Guide to learn more.

ENTRY TWO
PIE OF LIFE

———

Sometimes you need to step back from your
life and look down at it like you're
in a helicopter.

Sometimes it's hard to know why we do the things we do and feel the way we feel.

This is where the Pie of Life can really help. It's based on the insanely popular 'Wheel of Life' created by Paul J. Meyer. Used by millions of people across the world, this tool allows you to easily and quickly take a 'helicopter view' of your life as it is right now.

On the next page you'll find a big circle, divided into ten sections. These areas are the major categories of your life. I've provided some suggestions for you on the next page. But feel free to pick your own.

Once you've marked your categories onto each slice of the pie, it's time to score that slice. You are scoring each slice, based on your genuine satisfaction in that category. The points system is on a scale of zero to ten. Zero being the least amount of satisfaction and ten being the most. Move around the pie using a cross to mark your score on each line.

When you're done, join up the crosses. You should now have a really clear chart that maps out the core areas of your life. When you're done, try answering the Thought Triggers for this task.

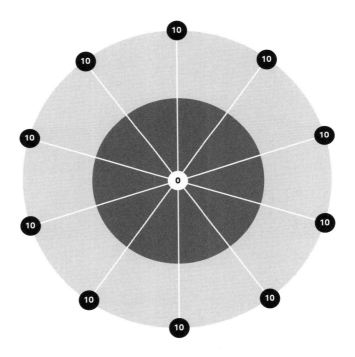

Suggested categories:
Work, Business, Career, Money, Health, Friends,
Family, Relationships, Fun, Home, Personal Growth,
Adventure, Happiness

HOW DID YOU SCORE?

**Why did you score each slice of the pie the way
you did? What scored the lowest? How could
you improve the score?**

_____

_____

_____

_____

_____

_____

_____

_____

_____

_____

_____

_____

_____

_____

_____

_____

_____

_____

**Make your Pie of Life as specific as you want.
You could make multiple pies for different
areas of your life.**

ENTRY THREE
TIME-STAMP

———

Today is a nice, easy session. You're just going to write about what you did today.

This exercise is similar to an ordinary 'diary' entry — summarising the day to day. But it's hugely important that we write this stuff down.

In fact psychologists have called the process of keeping a diary the 'Bridget Jones effect', taken from the terrible film with Renée Zellweger (just my opinion).

Leading psychologist, Matthew Lieberman, supports the idea through his recent research. He found that men benefited from writing about their experiences more that women. 'Men tend to show greater benefits and that is a bit counter-intuitive. But the reason might be that women more freely put their feelings into words, so this is less of a novel experience for them. For men it's more of a novelty.'

So just for a few seconds, step outside your comfort zone and summon your inner Bridget Jones. Today you're going to keep a diary. Use the Thought Triggers on the following page to guide you. And remember no one is going to read this, so try and be as frank and brutally honest as you can.

DESCRIBE YOUR DAY, TODAY

Time-stamp each activity and describe how each thing
you did, made you feel. Did you enjoy it? Why did you
do it? What would you have preferred to do?

HOW ARE YOU FEELING?

Circle, tick or cross out

stressed   nervous   tense   anxious   insecure   confused

positive   happy   hopeful   determined   glad   joyful   proud

bored   tired   hurt   angry   irritated   disappointed   annoyed

motivated   eager   excited   content   daring   safe   inspired

frustrated   furious   scared   trapped   worthless   unhappy

calm   grateful   strong   neutral   empathetic   mischievous   alive

regretful   upset   lonely   low   guilty   bitter   shocked   sad

confident   pleased   surprised   relieved   satisfied   energetic

Remember to take moments in your day to stop and
Check Yo' Self. Find out what I mean over on page
172 of the Support Guide.

ENTRY FOUR
YOUR ROLE

Being a guy these days involves a combination of roles. This exercise will get you looking at what you believe your role as a man is.

The role we play as men is changing right in front of us.

Now is a more important time than ever to reconnect with ourselves as men. And question what we believe our role to be.

We need to carve out our own roles. Discover our own ways to survive in the modern world. I believe the role of the modern-day man should be less defined, more open-minded and better connected to our emotions.

It's only society and our cultures that say we can't be sensitive, caring and self-aware. According to Tony Porter of TED Talk fame, what we've created over the years is the 'Man Box'. Filled with 'the ingredients of how we define what it means to be a man'. Things such as not crying, not expressing weakness or fear, demonstrating power (especially over women), not being like women, being tough and not needing help. And we're holding on to these and we need to learn to let them go.

Take the time to think about what you believe your role as a man has been throughout your life. And think about the kind of man you would like to be.

WHAT IS YOUR ROLE AS A MAN?

How does it feel to be a man? What is expected of you?
What kind of man would you like to be?

HOW ARE YOU FEELING?
Circle, tick or cross out

stressed · nervous · tense · anxious · insecure · confused
positive · happy · hopeful · determined · glad · joyful · proud
bored · tired · hurt · angry · irritated · disappointed · annoyed
motivated · eager · excited · content · daring · safe · inspired
frustrated · furious · scared · trapped · worthless · unhappy
calm · grateful · strong · neutral · empathetic · mischievous · alive
regretful · upset · lonely · low · guilty · bitter · shocked · sad
confident · pleased · surprised · relieved · satisfied · energetic

Try not to be too critical of yourself. This is a space
for you to reflect on the man you've become
and why.

ENTRY FIVE
GOOD VIBES

Most of us charge through our daily lives without really taking notice of the good stuff around us.

We just plough through time, hurtling towards the inevitable. Waking up, commuting, working, washing, shopping, sleeping and then repeating it all over again.

When was the last time you just stopped? Right there, in the middle of the street and just looked up and around you? Gazed in wonder at the clouds swirling above you or closed your eyes and just listened?

No matter how negative or stressed out you are, there will be something around you right now to appreciate. Something good to take in and absorb. You've just got to stop and look.

Studies have even been done by tons of professors and psychologists that show that being grateful for one thing everyday can improve not just your mental state but your physical too. Research also suggests that you'll sleep better, be healthier and exercise more as you'll have a proactive, positive attitude towards your life.

So embody your inner hippy. Peace and love man.

WHAT ARE YOU GRATEFUL FOR TODAY?

List all the things that you are grateful for. 'Cos not
everything sucks and you know it ...

HOW ARE YOU FEELING?

Circle, tick or cross out

(stressed) (nervous) (tense) (anxious) (insecure) (confused)
(positive) (happy) (hopeful) (determined) (glad) (joyful) (proud)
(bored) (tired) (hurt) (angry) (irritated) (disappointed) (annoyed)
(motivated) (eager) (excited) (content) (daring) (safe) (inspired)
(frustrated) (furious) (scared) (trapped) (worthless) (unhappy)
(calm) (grateful) (strong) (neutral) (empathetic) (mischievous) (alive)
(regretful) (upset) (lonely) (low) (guilty) (bitter) (shocked) (sad)
(confident) (pleased) (surprised) (relieved) (satisfied) (energetic)

For every bad thing in your day,
list five good things.

ENTRY SIX
HOME

The spaces you've made home and the places you've called home, have all moulded the person you've become.

'Where are you from?' is usually an easier question to answer, than 'where do you call home?'. But why?

When we were kids it was maybe an easier thing to answer. Because we believed home was where whoever was looking after us, was. But when we leave home, or get thrown out in my case, it's the people we really leave, not necessarily the space. The fact is, we can recreate that space anywhere, but not the people in it.

I believe 'home' is a combination of place and space. A place on a map, and the space around us. Be it a room, a house or a cardboard box. And it's how these two things evolve that play a role in the people we become.

Each time we move to a new place and create a new space, we change in some way. Find new things, meet new people and witness new experiences. Each one of those moves is a moment locked in time. Studies show that when we revisit these moments we tend to revert back to the people we once were. Not the people we've become since we left.

So home is one hell of a complex concept. And with it comes an abundance of memories and emotions. This will take you on a trip down memory lane, to get you to think about where you call home and why. It will ask you to reflect on where home is now, and what your dream home might be like.

WHERE DO YOU CALL HOME?

Think about where you've lived and how those places and
spaces made you feel. What made them feel like home?
Where do you feel most at home?

HOW ARE YOU FEELING?

Circle, tick or cross out

stressed · nervous · tense · anxious · insecure · confused
positive · happy · hopeful · determined · glad · joyful · proud
bored · tired · hurt · angry · irritated · disappointed · annoyed
motivated · eager · excited · content · daring · safe · inspired
frustrated · furious · scared · trapped · worthless · unhappy
calm · grateful · strong · neutral · empathetic · mischievous · alive
regretful · upset · lonely · low · guilty · bitter · shocked · sad
confident · pleased · surprised · relieved · satisfied · energetic

What would your dream home look like? Who would
be in it? Where would it be?

ENTRY SEVEN
BRAIN DUMP

Sometimes our heads get filled with noise and chatter. When this happens, things can get seriously exhausting.

The mixture of thoughts, sentences and emotions you're feeling need a place to live, other than in your head. And what better place to put them than in your journal.

Now there are lots of ways you can do this. But I suggest trying a Mind Map. They're insanely simple to do and mighty powerful.

You see our brains don't really work in a linear way. So lists don't necessarily perform that well. Our brains actually work a lot like maps. With lots of sprawling thoughts, ideas and emotions all connected to one another, each branching off to create even more connections and ideas. A Mind Map replicates this behaviour. Just in a more visual way.

To create a Mind Map, stick a core thought in the middle of the page. Now draw a line from the middle and write down something based on that central idea, then circle it. And then keep repeating until you're exhausted and there is no space left on the page.

If you need help with this task head to www.mindjournals.com to download a more detailed worksheet.

_____

WHAT'S ON YOUR MIND?

List all the things on your mind. Good or bad, jobs
or chores, upcoming events. Absolutely everything
you can think of.

HOW ARE YOU FEELING?

Circle, tick or cross out

stressed) (nervous) (tense) (anxious) (insecure) (confused

positive) (happy) (hopeful) (determined) (glad) (joyful) (proud

bored) (tired) (hurt) (angry) (irritated) (disappointed) (annoyed

motivated) (eager) (excited) (content) (daring) (safe) (inspired

frustrated) (furious) (scared) (trapped) (worthless) (unhappy

calm) (grateful) (strong) (neutral) (empathetic) (mischievous) (alive

regretful) (upset) (lonely) (low) (guilty) (bitter) (shocked) (sad

confident) (pleased) (surprised) (relieved) (satisfied) (energetic

Do this task however you feel. Just unleash those
thoughts on the page and keep going until you
have nothing left.

ENTRY EIGHT
GOOD TIMES

The good times should always outweigh the
bad times. This exercise will help tip
the scales in your favour.

It's a fact that time flies when you're having fun. And drags when you're not.

It's simply because, when we're having fun our brains are distracted. Even though you might be doing a single activity, your mind is firing off multiple emotions and thoughts. And is less focused on a single thing such as time.

That's why when we're bored we clock-watch. Agonising over every minute. It's not actually going any slower. Time is a constant. It never increases or decreases. Only our attention to it does.

This all has an effect on how we approach new activities. Our minds hold on to bad experiences more easily than good. So if you're doing something that is dragging on and you're not enjoying it, you're more likely to remember it. And not want to do it, or something similar again.

Studies suggest that in order to improve your own happiness you need to look back at good times. Relive them in your mind and experience all those positive emotions. The idea is that by doing this you will learn to remember the good times more than the bad. And your brain will react in a positive way, making you think that time is flying. Try it next time you're bored out of your mind.

In this exercise you're going to focus on a specific time when you had fun. And you're going to enjoy every minute of it. Today's session is going to fly.

THE MOST FUN YOU'VE EVER HAD?

Choose a time in your life that you had the most fun. Why was it so good? Who were you with? Where were you? How could you relive that moment?

HOW ARE YOU FEELING?

Circle, tick or cross out

stressed nervous tense anxious insecure confused
positive happy hopeful determined glad joyful proud
bored tired hurt angry irritated disappointed annoyed
motivated eager excited content daring safe inspired
frustrated furious scared trapped worthless unhappy
calm grateful strong neutral empathetic mischievous alive
regretful upset lonely low guilty bitter shocked sad
confident pleased surprised relieved satisfied energetic

When times are bad, time travel back to this moment. Relive it. Having fun is essential to your health and well-being, remember that.

ENTRY NINE
WORK

———

When you love your job, it's no longer a job.
It's a hobby that you get paid to do. Sadly
most of us don't work like this.

Our jobs take up so much of our lives. We spend hours and hours each day grafting, leaving not much time for anything else.

And that's great if your job makes you feel good. But not so great if your job sucks the life out of you.

Sometimes the discomfort we feel in our jobs is a result of our jobs not representing who we are as individuals. The person we are in the workplace, may not be the person we are deep down. Or we feel the work we are doing doesn't actually fit with our core beliefs or interests. When this happens, our jobs suck. And that means for 8 hours everyday, our life sucks.

It doesn't have to be this way. You do have a choice. Two very simple choices. You can leave and find a job you love. Or if that's not an option — double up on all the good things in your life. Do the things that bring you joy and happiness, twice as much.

We all get busy being busy, that we don't often get the time to stand back and review our jobs. Not based on output, money or time — but on how they make us feel. Use this exercise as your review time.

DO YOU LOVE WHAT YOU DO?

What would you change about your career so far? What
advice would you give others? If work sucks, how
could you balance this out?

HOW ARE YOU FEELING?

Circle, tick or cross out

stressed) (nervous) (tense) (anxious) (insecure) (confused

positive) (happy) (hopeful) (determined) (glad) (joyful) (proud

bored) (tired) (hurt) (angry) (irritated) (disappointed) (annoyed

motivated) (eager) (excited) (content) (daring) (safe) (inspired

frustrated) (furious) (scared) (trapped) (worthless) (unhappy

calm) (grateful) (strong) (neutral) (empathetic) (mischievous) (alive

regretful) (upset) (lonely) (low) (guilty) (bitter) (shocked) (sad

confident) (pleased) (surprised) (relieved) (satisfied) (energetic

Student or unemployed? If so what would you like
from having a career? What goals do you have in
mind? What would be your dream job?

ENTRY TEN
RAP BATTLE

If you ever want to feel super motivated, and ready to take on anything, you need to fill your eardrums with some hip-hop.

Rappers are the dons of writing a journal. In fact, there's quite a lot you can learn from hip-hop music.

So much so that two researchers from Cambridge University have found that hip-hop can help with a range of issues from depression to schizophrenia.

The power of hip-hop comes from rap artists using their lyrics to draw you picture of what they're going through. They openly pen all their hardships and emotions down on paper and then repeat them over a beat, through a microphone, for you to listen to.

Their rags to riches stories inspire a huge range of listeners. From homeless kids, to business execs. They create a message that other people can relate to. When they rap about their struggles, it strikes a chord with listeners and reminds them that they're not alone. When those same rappers, rap about success, it makes you feel that you too can make it out of whatever bad situation you feel you're in.

Writing rap lyrics is a therapeutic tool for self discovery and growth. As it's no different to writing an entry in your journal. Most rap artists begin all their raps, by writing down lyrics in a book. Like you're about to do. They turn all their troubles and ambitions into powerful pieces of spoken word.

But it all begins as an entry. A page in their journal of life, spoken through their music. Now it's your turn to write your life as a rap.

WRITE A RAP ABOUT YOUR LIFE

Think of the greatest rappers and poets of
your time and try writing your own rhyme
about your life.

HOW ARE YOU FEELING?

Circle, tick or cross out

stressed · nervous · tense · anxious · insecure · confused

positive · happy · hopeful · determined · glad · joyful · proud

bored · tired · hurt · angry · irritated · disappointed · annoyed

motivated · eager · excited · content · daring · safe · inspired

frustrated · furious · scared · trapped · worthless · unhappy

calm · grateful · strong · neutral · empathetic · mischievous · alive

regretful · upset · lonely · low · guilty · bitter · shocked · sad

confident · pleased · surprised · relieved · satisfied · energetic

If it helps, try listening to some hip-hop or reading
some poetry to help get you in the zone.

IT'S OK TO CHANGE DIRECTION.

SOMETIMES YOU HAVE TO BE LOST BEFORE YOU CAN FIND YOUR WAY.

STAGE TWO
HURDLES

2

First off — bravo man. High fives all round. You've completed the Warm Up stage and you should feel pretty damn good about yourself.

Now we're going to step it up a gear. This new set of Thought Triggers are going to test you a bit more than the first. In order to build strength you've got to push yourself harder. Don't be afraid of failing this. Cos' you can't. It's impossible to get wrong.

This next stage is all about you and the people around you. I really want you to think about how these people have shaped the person you've become.

We're also going to dig a bit deeper into what makes you tick. How you cope with certain things such as fear, anger and stress. At the moment you might be trying to move forward and these hurdles are in your way. Or you might be flying through but keep catching your heel on the tip of the hurdle you're jumping. Either way this stage will get your mind thinking more clearly, allowing you to focus on the next hurdle.

This is all part of the training. All part of getting your mind fit so you can tackle the big workouts in the final stage.

So let's crack on with the next exercise.

ENTRY ELEVEN
RELATIONSHIP MAP

———

In order to look at ourselves, sometimes we need to look at the people around us. And question why they're there and how we value them.

In order for us to find out who's really important in our lives, we need to map out all the people that are in it.

To do this simply, you're going to put down all the key people in your life on the Relationship Map on the next page. It's a hugely effective exercise that allows you to create a clear picture of the people around you. It gives you a moment to pause and think of how you value each of them.

From doing this you'll start to see patterns in your relationships. Highlighting people who you thought were close to you but are not that close at all. And most importantly how you value yourself out of all the people you've mapped out.

Something I've learned from doing this is that it's easy to lose yourself to others. To neglect your own needs and make others more important than yourself. Sometimes it can happen without you even noticing. Let this exercise be your marker.

On the next page, plot all the key people in your life. Then list those people in numerical order from 1 to however many people you wrote down. Who ever is at number 1 is the most important.

The key point though, is where you are on that list ...

You

1.	6.	11.
2.	7.	12.
3.	8.	13.
4.	9.	14.
5.	10.	15.

WHERE ARE YOU?

What patterns emerged? Who was at number 1 and why?
How did you value yourself?

You could use a Mind Map approach or create
rings around yourself representing inner and
outer circles.

ENTRY TWELVE
ROLE MODELS

Role models can be pretty powerful beings.
They can have a huge impact on our lives,
helping us to become even better
versions of ourselves.

Growing up we probably all had role models at some point.

They might have been your father, a teacher, a sportsman or even a superhero. But as we grow into adults, our perceptions of these role models might change. Our heroes are no longer heroes. We either no longer need them or our view of them has changed. And this can be tough to deal with and leave us feeling lost.

Having a role model in your life is a key part of self-improvement.

There's a great quote by the Irish novelist, Oliver Goldsmith, that says 'People seldom improve when they have no other model but themselves to copy.'

I think this is so true. And what I've found massively helpful is to have role models that focus on the specific goals I'm trying to achieve. Be it in my health or in my work.

Research suggests that people have a better chance of achieving their goals if they pick a role model that aligns more closely with their desired outcome.

With this in mind, try and think about the role models you've had in your life and how they've influenced you.

WHO ARE YOUR ROLE MODELS?

Are they the same as when you were a kid? How have they changed? Who would make a good role model now?

HOW ARE YOU FEELING?

Circle, tick or cross out

(stressed) (nervous) (tense) (anxious) (insecure) (confused)
(positive) (happy) (hopeful) (determined) (glad) (joyful) (proud)
(bored) (tired) (hurt) (angry) (irritated) (disappointed) (annoyed)
(motivated) (eager) (excited) (content) (daring) (safe) (inspired)
(frustrated) (furious) (scared) (trapped) (worthless) (unhappy)
(calm) (grateful) (strong) (neutral) (empathetic) (mischievous) (alive)
(regretful) (upset) (lonely) (low) (guilty) (bitter) (shocked) (sad)
(confident) (pleased) (surprised) (relieved) (satisfied) (energetic)

If you're struggling to think of a new role model, look at your goal from entry 1 and find someone who's achieved it.

ENTRY THIRTEEN
SUPERPOWERS

———

Some strengths we're just born with. Others are formed by confronting our deepest and darkest weaknesses.

We all have our strengths, a set of superpowers that are unique to us.

Sometimes though, our strengths are buried within our weaknesses. A part of ourselves that we're not big fans of.

Take Bruce Banner for example, he doesn't really like getting angry. But his weakness gives him his superpower to become the Hulk. The giant green beast that can smash through anything and defeat the toughest of enemies.

We shouldn't look at our weaknesses as negatives. As all of our weaknesses can become strengths. Our weaknesses cloud our true strengths. Our weaknesses are bound to us through fear. We're afraid of what makes us weak. But breaking through this fear can lead to a power so strong, it completely changes the fabric of who we are.

Our weaknesses make us feel vulnerable. But being vulnerable isn't a sign of weakness. It's a sign of strength. This is why you shouldn't look at your weaknesses as negative things. Weaknesses are just strengths you've not harnessed yet.

WHAT'S YOUR SUPERPOWER?

What's your greatest strength & biggest weakness? What one weakness could become a new superpower? What would it take to unleash that new superpower?

HOW ARE YOU FEELING?

Circle, tick or cross out

stressed   nervous   tense   anxious   insecure   confused

positive   happy   hopeful   determined   glad   joyful   proud

bored   tired   hurt   angry   irritated   disappointed   annoyed

motivated   eager   excited   content   daring   safe   inspired

frustrated   furious   scared   trapped   worthless   unhappy

calm   grateful   strong   neutral   empathetic   mischievous   alive

regretful   upset   lonely   low   guilty   bitter   shocked   sad

confident   pleased   surprised   relieved   satisfied   energetic

Weaknesses aren't bad or negative things.
Remember that.

ENTRY FOURTEEN
RELATIONSHIPS

Pause for a moment and reflect on all the relationships you've had in your life. Not just with people but with yourself and the world around you.

The ones you've had, the one's you've got — from the healthy, to the not so healthy.

We have relationships with so many things and so many people these days. We're constantly wired in to a connection with someone or something. And through all these connections we build relationships. From our partners, parents, colleagues and random people on the commute, to devices, food, sex and money.

Relationship overload.

Take this moment to unplug from the connections and reflect on just a couple of your key relationships. It could be with your partner, your job or your family. Or your relationship with porn, bad food or money.

The importance of all of this is to explore why you have these relationships. The positives and the negatives. Studies have shown that the relationships we have come from our early connections in life. When we were kids. Connections we made with the people, environment and objects around us in those first few years.

So pick a couple of key relationships that you've experienced and take the time to reflect on what you've learned from them.

REFLECT ON YOUR RELATIONSHIPS

Positive and negative. How have these had an impact on your life? What have you learned from them?

HOW ARE YOU FEELING?

Circle, tick or cross out

stressed · nervous · tense · anxious · insecure · confused
positive · happy · hopeful · determined · glad · joyful · proud
bored · tired · hurt · angry · irritated · disappointed · annoyed
motivated · eager · excited · content · daring · safe · inspired
frustrated · furious · scared · trapped · worthless · unhappy
calm · grateful · strong · neutral · empathetic · mischievous · alive
regretful · upset · lonely · low · guilty · bitter · shocked · sad
confident · pleased · surprised · relieved · satisfied · energetic

Finding this one tough? Try using your Relationship Map as a starting point.

ENTRY FIFTEEN
FEAR FEEDS FEAR

And sometimes it's easy to find things to feed it. This exercise will help you starve the beast.

Anxiety is a common symptom of fear. As are panic attacks. Both of which I suffer from. And in totally irrational situations. Such as train rides.

Growing up, I lived with fear day in day out. Most days were filled with 'what if' scenarios. Worrying about what condition I might come home and find mum in. All this 'what if' thinking is exactly what drives my anxiety. The fear of 'what if'.

Over the years I've learned to retrain my brain to try and let go of these fears. They still pop up now and again, in completely irrational situations. In fact most of our fears tend to be irrational. What we believe to be the worst outcome, never really transpires. Yet we still feed the fear beast. And the more we feed it, the more it grows and the more power it gains. A vicious cycle ensues.

Fear is one of the most powerful and primitive of human emotions. It alerts us to danger. Both emotionally and physically. In fact a study in the 1970s found that the mind allocates more space and energy to fear, than to any other emotion. So we naturally hold on to it.

But you can let go of fear. You can, like I've learned, retrain your brain into learning there is no real threat. To do this you need to prove to your mind that there is nothing to fear, by doing the exact thing you're afraid of.

WHAT'S YOUR BIGGEST FEAR?

Describe how this fear makes you feel... How do you manage this fear? Does it prevent you from doing certain things? How could you confront this fear?

HOW ARE YOU FEELING?

Circle, tick or cross out

stressed · nervous · tense · anxious · insecure · confused
positive · happy · hopeful · determined · glad · joyful · proud
bored · tired · hurt · angry · irritated · disappointed · annoyed
motivated · eager · excited · content · daring · safe · inspired
frustrated · furious · scared · trapped · worthless · unhappy
calm · grateful · strong · neutral · empathetic · mischievous · alive
regretful · upset · lonely · low · guilty · bitter · shocked · sad
confident · pleased · surprised · relieved · satisfied · energetic

Find fear, hunt it down, look it in the
eyes and say fuck you.

ENTRY SIXTEEN
STRESS BUCKET

When there's loads of stuff doing your head in, it's sometimes hard to know what's causing you to feel so stressed out.

You can only tackle your stress when you know exactly what is stressing you out.

So how do you locate the sources of your stress? Simple, draw your Stress Bucket. The Stress Bucket is a tool created by leading psychologists, Alison Brabban and Douglas Turkington. And it's hugely effective at nailing what's really stressing you out, and how the way you're dealing with it is having an effect on you.

Everyone has a different size bucket, depending on how much stress they can carry. Yours might be small or it could be huge. Either way buckets contain water and water equals stress. And how many things are stressing you out determines how full your bucket it is.

The Stress Bucket has a little tap at the bottom though, like a keg of beer. Every time you look after yourself and do something that relieves your stress, water is let out of it. The less you look after yourself, the less the tap opens. And the fuller the bucket gets.

Use the Stress Bucket diagram on the next page to find all the things that are causing you to feel stressed. Draw a water line on the bucket to mark where your current stress level is. And at the bottom where the little tap is, write down all the things that you do to look after yourself and help relieve your stress.

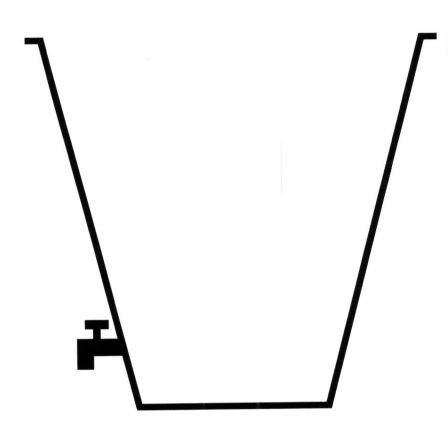

WHAT'S IN YOUR STRESS BUCKET?

Where is your current stress level? How do you cope with your stress? And how could you cope with it better?

_____

_____

_____

_____

_____

_____

_____

_____

_____

_____

_____

_____

_____

_____

_____

_____

_____

_____

_____

Once you've done this session, head to the back of the book and read Stress Test on page 174.

ENTRY SEVENTEEN
ANGER MOTHERFU*KER

Anger is a tough emotion to deal with because it's an instinctive response to pain. Either caused by ourselves or someone else.

Being angry at the people we love is not easy.

I was full of rage at my mum when she died. But I found it easier to get angry with the door not shutting or the TV remote not working, than with her. And how could I get angry with her anyway, she wasn't here anymore. However, locking up my anger only led to more frustration and more anger. I needed to let it out. And that's where, for me, journaling really helped.

Studies have shown that suppressing your anger could be seriously bad for your body as well as your mind. In fact it could be as bad for you as smoking. So it's super important to get that anger and negative energy out.

The longer you hold on to it, the more you'll feel tense, irritable and liable to snap. And when that happens, things get broken, people get hurt and you'll end up feeling even worse.

Letting it out to the guy that cuts you up on the highway can end up getting you arrested. So do the right thing and use this journal like I did, as a safe place to let rip.

Take five and give the paper some verbal abuse.

WHAT MAKES YOU ANGRY?

Describe what happened the last time you got angry. What made you angry? How did you feel before, during and after? How do you deal with your anger?

HOW ARE YOU FEELING?

Circle, tick or cross out

stressed · nervous · tense · anxious · insecure · confused
positive · happy · hopeful · determined · glad · joyful · proud
bored · tired · hurt · angry · irritated · disappointed · annoyed
motivated · eager · excited · content · daring · safe · inspired
frustrated · furious · scared · trapped · worthless · unhappy
calm · grateful · strong · neutral · empathetic · mischievous · alive
regretful · upset · lonely · low · guilty · bitter · shocked · sad
confident · pleased · surprised · relieved · satisfied · energetic

Scream. Shout. Yell.
Just let the anger out — safely.
Violence doesn't lead to anywhere good.

ENTRY EIGHTEEN
EVEN THUGS CRY

———

I've always found it hard to cry. It's just never been something I've felt comfortable doing. But crying is in fact a very manly thing to do.

Back in the day, men that cried were seen as strong masculine figures. It showed others that they cared and had integrity.

Abraham Lincoln was an emotional chap, who famously showed his tears to convey his passion and honesty for the things he believed in.

And while in today's culture guys still struggle to cry out of fear of being judged, research suggests that we are returning to the belief that crying is a sign of strength. Tests carried out on football players showed that players who cried after a game, no matter the result, had higher levels of self-esteem. And this evident in a lot of top flight sportsmen.

Now don't get me wrong there's a time and place to cry. A combat soldier on the battlefield can't stop to cry. Emergency service responders also have to suppress their tears and remain calm in the most extreme situations. But this is why it's super important to learn how to un-suppress those hard-earned tears.

Don't be afraid to shed them. Learn to use the things that make you cry to your advantage. Save them for a later date. Keep them in your toolbox. Don't feel ashamed — it doesn't make you weak or less of a man.

HOW DOES CRYING MAKE YOU FEEL?

Think about the last time you shed a tear — what was it over?
What's your relationship with crying? When do you feel
it's acceptable to cry?

HOW ARE YOU FEELING?

Circle, tick or cross out

stressed | nervous | tense | anxious | insecure | confused

positive | happy | hopeful | determined | glad | joyful | proud

bored | tired | hurt | angry | irritated | disappointed | annoyed

motivated | eager | excited | content | daring | safe | inspired

frustrated | furious | scared | trapped | worthless | unhappy

calm | grateful | strong | neutral | empathetic | mischievous | alive

regretful | upset | lonely | low | guilty | bitter | shocked | sad

confident | pleased | surprised | relieved | satisfied | energetic

Crying doesn't make you weak.
It's OK to grab the Kleenex Man-size.

ENTRY NINETEEN
BURY THE HATCHET

Holding on to bad feelings towards other people can leave you feeling crap.

Holding on to bad feelings towards other people can leave you feeling crap.

In fact research shows that holding a grudge can take a toll on your mind and body. When someone wrongs us, we often experience anger and stress. And the longer we don't forgive, the longer we hold on to these feelings.

Letting go of this stuff and focusing on forgiveness releases the tension in your body. Forgiveness is not about becoming best buddies with whoever harmed you. Our brains don't work like that — we can't just forgive and then forget.

Forgiveness is a constant exercise.

Finding forgiveness is not easy though, especially when the person who hurt you is someone you care about. It's even harder when the person you need to forgive is yourself. To move from anger to forgiveness you need to get this stuff out.

Today's exercise will allow you to get it out and start the process of letting go and accepting that what happened — happened.

WHO WOULD YOU LIKE TO FORGIVE?

How does holding a grudge against someone make you feel?
Are you ready to forgive them? What would you
say to them if you had the chance?

HOW ARE YOU FEELING?

Circle, tick or cross out

stressed   nervous   tense   anxious   insecure   confused

positive   happy   hopeful   determined   glad   joyful   proud

bored   tired   hurt   angry   irritated   disappointed   annoyed

motivated   eager   excited   content   daring   safe   inspired

frustrated   furious   scared   trapped   worthless   unhappy

calm   grateful   strong   neutral   empathetic   mischievous   alive

regretful   upset   lonely   low   guilty   bitter   shocked   sad

confident   pleased   surprised   relieved   satisfied   energetic

What things have you done that you feel bad
about? It's OK to forgive yourself — how could
you do this?

ENTRY TWENTY
PEN PAL

We no longer write letters. We write emails.
And we write way too many of them. So today,
let's write to someone. Don't worry though,
we're not going to send it.

A physical letter is a powerful tool. It uses what I've been banging on about throughout this entire book — getting your thoughts down on paper.

You can use this exercise in a number of ways. From telling someone how you really feel (good or bad), to writing to yourself as you are now want to be in the future.

Writing a letter is such an incredible thing to do because it creates a non-verbal dialogue. It's hard to put your thoughts and feelings into words. It's why you're giving this journal a go. Letter writing turns everything you're experiencing internally, into an actual conversation.

I've written tons of letters over the years in my journal. To myself, to my mum, to partners, ex-partners, business partners, family members and even to the universe. And they range from asking for help to telling them what's on my mind. The ones I write to myself, are mostly reminders that everything will be OK.

Remember you're not sending this letter. In fact I've never sent any of the letters I've ever written. The point is not in sending them. But in the process of writing them.

WHO WOULD YOU WRITE A LETTER TO?

Write a letter to someone, past or present. What do you want to tell them? Is there something you wish you could tell them but are too afraid to say?

HOW ARE YOU FEELING?

Circle, tick or cross out

stressed · nervous · tense · anxious · insecure · confused
positive · happy · hopeful · determined · glad · joyful · proud
bored · tired · hurt · angry · irritated · disappointed · annoyed
motivated · eager · excited · content · daring · safe · inspired
frustrated · furious · scared · trapped · worthless · unhappy
calm · grateful · strong · neutral · empathetic · mischievous · alive
regretful · upset · lonely · low · guilty · bitter · shocked · sad
confident · pleased · surprised · relieved · satisfied · energetic

Be honest and be frank. This is where you can tell them anything and everything. You've got this.

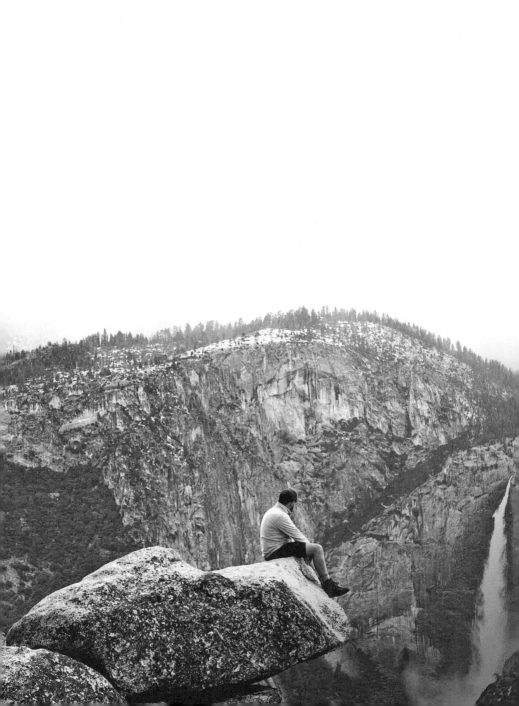

WHEN WE
EXPERIENCE AN
ADVENTURE IT'S
NOT A NEW PLACE
WE FIND.

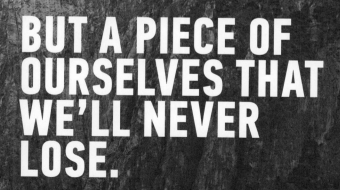

BUT A PIECE OF
OURSELVES THAT
WE'LL NEVER
LOSE.

STAGE THREE
STRENGTH

Hold. The. Phone. Let's just take a second to see how far you've come. Flick through your journal from the beginning to here. You wrote all that stuff — that is some epic shit.

And, since you breezed through the last section so easily, I've made this final section a bit tougher.

You're going to come across some tricky Thought Triggers over the next few pages. Some of them you might not feel ready to respond to. But you can and you will. You've already done 20 of these now.

This is like the last 10 reps in a workout or the last 10 laps to the finishing line. Just stay focused and pace yourself. This is where core strength is gained so remember to rest well too.

If you're struggling at any point, then just keep reading the Thought Trigger over a period of days. Sit with it, allow it to sink in. The response will come and if it doesn't, well then write that down. Explain why you can't answer it.

This final stage is all about your future, your needs and what's important to you. It will only work if you're completely honest with yourself. A journal is like a letterbox. If you only post bullshit, then that's all you'll ever read and you won't learn anything of value. Post only what is true, what is meaningful and what truly matters to you.

You can do this. So go do it.

ENTRY TWENTY-ONE
FUCK IT

The Fuck It List will help take all the things you think are important but really aren't and learn to say 'Fuck It' instead.

We give too much importance to the mundane things in our lives.

This importance then gives them power over us and we're soon at their mercy. Sometimes it could be people, but mostly it's tasks, or things we feel we should do. This is why it's the opposite to a Bucket List.

A Bucket List is a list of all the things you want to do. And a Fuck It List is all the things you don't want to do. And in order to have an effective Bucket List, you need a solid Fuck It List.

But there is a whole other side to a Fuck It List. And this is to embrace the mindset of 'giving less fucks' about certain things in life — as the 'Fuck It' pioneer, Mark Mason would say. His insanely popular articles and best-selling book 'The Subtle Art of Not Giving a Fuck' supports the concept behind the Fuck It List.

It's not about not caring. In fact it's about caring more. But only about the things that are truly important to you. And less about the things that are not. It's a mindset. It's a way to approach situations and problems. Don't give the things that are doing your head in any more power or time. Learn to not give a fuck about them instead.

WHAT'S ON YOUR FUCK IT LIST?

Write down all the things you would like to say 'Fuck It' to. How could you stick to the list and make sure they don't get done? How does the Fuck It List make you feel?

HOW ARE YOU FEELING?

Circle, tick or cross out

stressed   nervous   tense   anxious   insecure   confused

positive   happy   hopeful   determined   glad   joyful   proud

bored   tired   hurt   angry   irritated   disappointed   annoyed

motivated   eager   excited   content   daring   safe   inspired

frustrated   furious   scared   trapped   worthless   unhappy

calm   grateful   strong   neutral   empathetic   mischievous   alive

regretful   upset   lonely   low   guilty   bitter   shocked   sad

confident   pleased   surprised   relieved   satisfied   energetic

There might have been a time in your life, where you truly thought 'Fuck It'. If so when was it and what made you not give a fuck anymore?

ENTRY TWENTY-TWO
JUST SAY NO

The word Yes is so much easier to use than the word No. But learning to say No can lead to more meaningful Yes's.

We believe that Yes is a positive and No is a negative. This is all balls.

Whilst I'm all for grabbing life by the earlobes and saying Yes, I'm also bang up for a bit of balance. You can't say Yes to everything. You can't sacrifice your own needs and wants, if that's where answering Yes leads to. And I've made this mistake time and time again. In work, love and life. Said Yes, when I really meant No.

Saying No is about setting ground rules for yourself. And giving yourself the strength to not negotiate with others. There's a huge psychological cost to saying Yes when really you mean No. And even though we perceive it as a negative word, filled with negative repercussions, it is in fact saying Yes that could to lead to a negative outcome.

No is a power word. Those that use it show strength. Leading psychologist on the matter, Adam Grant, says that, 'the ability to say No is one of the most important skills one can have'.

Saying No is not easy though. And people will fight and challenge your response. But this is their issue and not yours. If saying No is truly how you feel, people can't argue with you. Because you can never be wrong if you're just being honest about how you feel.

LEARN TO SAY NO

Who and what do you find hard saying no to? Why is this?
How does saying no make you feel? What for you
is non-negotiable?

HOW ARE YOU FEELING?

Circle, tick or cross out

stressed　nervous　tense　anxious　insecure　confused
positive　happy　hopeful　determined　glad　joyful　proud
bored　tired　hurt　angry　irritated　disappointed　annoyed
motivated　eager　excited　content　daring　safe　inspired
frustrated　furious　scared　trapped　worthless　unhappy
calm　grateful　strong　neutral　empathetic　mischievous　alive
regretful　upset　lonely　low　guilty　bitter　shocked　sad
confident　pleased　surprised　relieved　satisfied　energetic

It takes a lot of bravery to learn to say No.
If you're struggling turn to page 176 to
learn more about saying No.

ENTRY TWENTY-THREE
PASTIME

Don't ever underestimate the power of a pastime. It can really improve every part of your life. Here's how.

It's important to do the things you love, that bring you joy and happiness.

Some people call these things a hobby. And not having one, probably means you're working too hard.

It's super important to create some balance and get some fun time in to your day-to-day life. Even the doc approves the idea of having a hobby in your life. Dr Kevin Eschleman, a professor at the San Francisco State University calls the hobby effect 'recovery from work'. And his fascinating research shows how effective and important creative hobbies are to our performance in day-to-day life.

They have the power to lead to some awesome outcomes. Like meeting new people, building confidence, relieving stress, making you more productive, avoiding boredom, keeping you feeling young and giving you a more positive outlook on life.

Use this exercise as an opportunity to explore some ideas for what hobbies you might enjoy trying. And if you already have a hobby, use this space to find a new one and express how your current hobby affects your life.

Date:

WHAT BRINGS YOU JOY?

What activity do you love doing but rarely get the opportunity to do? When are you truly happy and time disappears?

HOW ARE YOU FEELING?

Circle, tick or cross out

stressed · nervous · tense · anxious · insecure · confused

positive · happy · hopeful · determined · glad · joyful · proud

bored · tired · hurt · angry · irritated · disappointed · annoyed

motivated · eager · excited · content · daring · safe · inspired

frustrated · furious · scared · trapped · worthless · unhappy

calm · grateful · strong · neutral · empathetic · mischievous · alive

regretful · upset · lonely · low · guilty · bitter · shocked · sad

confident · pleased · surprised · relieved · satisfied · energetic

If you can't think of a hobby, try listing all the things you'd like to try. Then make a plan to test them all out. Go have some fun.

ENTRY TWENTY-FOUR
MAKE TOMORROW TODAY

——

Stop putting things off. It's really not doing
you any good. Shit's not getting done, you feel
crap and so do the people around you. In this
session you're going to stop delaying things.

We all put things off. It's not because we don't want to do them. We just don't feel like doing them. And we're happy to wait until we do.

Some might call this procrastination. And Professor Joseph Ferrari, a leading psychologist on the matter, has research to support the claim that nearly 20% of Americans are chronic procrastinators.

In fact if there was one way to succeed in not succeeding in life, it would be to fall victim to procrastination. It's like a virus. It feeds on its host. On your own self-doubt and fear.

The scary thing is that sometimes we're oblivious to the fact that we're even doing it. We trick ourselves into thinking that the logical step to being productive is to avoid other tasks.

This task is all about becoming aware of what you're avoiding. What you're constantly putting off, and how you can focus on it.

Try to focus on how good you're going to feel once you've ticked this thing off your list. And remember to reward yourself when you've completed it — bribe yourself with something fun.

Lastly don't forget to ask for help. I don't mean, getting someone else to do it for you. But asking with help to get it done. Making it public will also lead to a greater chance of you getting it done, as it will add a healthy dose of motivation.

Date:

STOP PUTTING THIS OFF

What's the one thing you're always putting off? What's stopping you from doing it? What needs to be done to achieve it? How will you do it?

HOW ARE YOU FEELING?

Circle, tick or cross out

stressed   nervous   tense   anxious   insecure   confused
positive   happy   hopeful   determined   glad   joyful   proud
bored   tired   hurt   angry   irritated   disappointed   annoyed
motivated   eager   excited   content   daring   safe   inspired
frustrated   furious   scared   trapped   worthless   unhappy
calm   grateful   strong   neutral   empathetic   mischievous   alive
regretful   upset   lonely   low   guilty   bitter   shocked   sad
confident   pleased   surprised   relieved   satisfied   energetic

Use this exercise to release all that pent-up hesitation. And then go do it. I dare you.

ENTRY TWENTY-FIVE
TIME TO DAYDREAM

Unlock your true potential, the unrestricted version of yourself, free from fears and doubts, all in the comfort of your own dream world.

Martin Luther King had a dream. He allowed himself the freedom to dream about something he believed to be possible.

He visualised it in his mind's eye. He pictured the future of the world to be different. And while I'm not here to argue if his dream came true or not. His dream sparked an entire movement. Evidence that dreaming can be powerful in leading to change.

There's been a huge amount of work done by a large number of professors as to the benefits of daydreaming. Eric Klinger a top professor in the field of dreams (no, not the Kevin Costner movie, even though that's about living out your dreams too) has found that daydreaming can give your brain a boost in power and strength. 'It's an essential resource for coping with life', he says in his research.

Daydreaming is one of the most common and profound things we do as human beings. It allows us to time travel into the future. To write our own stories of how we want our lives to unfold. We forget our fears, envisage our truest desires and picture the success of achieving our goals. Daydreaming is just pre-planning. If our thoughts are real, our dreams can be too.

Use today's exercise to allow yourself to daydream and then record that dream. Embrace your own freedom and imagination.

WHAT DO YOU DREAM OF?

How would you spend your time, if money wasn't an issue?
What would you like the story of your life to be like? What did
you dream of doing when you were a kid?

HOW ARE YOU FEELING?

Circle, tick or cross out

(stressed) (nervous) (tense) (anxious) (insecure) (confused)
(positive) (happy) (hopeful) (determined) (glad) (joyful) (proud)
(bored) (tired) (hurt) (angry) (irritated) (disappointed) (annoyed)
(motivated) (eager) (excited) (content) (daring) (safe) (inspired)
(frustrated) (furious) (scared) (trapped) (worthless) (unhappy)
(calm) (grateful) (strong) (neutral) (empathetic) (mischievous) (alive)
(regretful) (upset) (lonely) (low) (guilty) (bitter) (shocked) (sad)
(confident) (pleased) (surprised) (relieved) (satisfied) (energetic)

Close your eyes, sit quietly and really immerse
yourself in your dream. Picture every little detail,
every thought and feeling. And then record it here.

ENTRY TWENTY-SIX
MISSING IN ACTION

Life is rarely complete. And at times we can feel lost and confused about where we are, what we're doing and where we're going.

We fill our lives with so many objectives and missions. But how do we really know if the things we're doing are the things we really want to do?

Simple. Find what's missing.

In today's exercise you're going to explore the areas of your life that might be missing something. It could be purpose, passion, meaning, fun or even adventure. All of which, according to some of the world's greatest thinkers, doers and explorers — create the foundations of a happy and fulfilling life.

Take adventure for example. Something that was abundant in our childhoods that has slowly disappeared as we've got older and grown into stressed-out adults. When we experience an adventure what we actually find is not a new skill, or a new place on the map, it's a piece of ourselves that we'll never lose.

Don't start with where you are. Start with where you're not. Face the feeling of being lost. Find a part of your life that is missing something. It will lead you to some profound answers and maybe take you on your own adventure.

_____

WHAT'S MISSING FROM YOUR LIFE?

Is it a sense of purpose, passion, meaning, fun or even adventure? What could you do to find more of these things in your life? What's holding you back from finding them?

HOW ARE YOU FEELING?

Circle, tick or cross out

stressed   nervous   tense   anxious   insecure   confused

positive   happy   hopeful   determined   glad   joyful   proud

bored   tired   hurt   angry   irritated   disappointed   annoyed

motivated   eager   excited   content   daring   safe   inspired

frustrated   furious   scared   trapped   worthless   unhappy

calm   grateful   strong   neutral   empathetic   mischievous   alive

regretful   upset   lonely   low   guilty   bitter   shocked   sad

confident   pleased   surprised   relieved   satisfied   energetic

After writing today, reward yourself. Do something you love doing. Check out page 178 in the Support Guide to remind yourself why.

ENTRY TWENTY-SEVEN
BUCKET LIST 100

This exercise is like your bog standard
Bucket List on steroids. It's not meant to be
completed in a single session, it's meant to
last an entire lifetime.

This is a challenge to yourself to think of 100 things you could with your time on this planet.

Think of this list as your top 100 things to do. Try thinking about others, as well as yourself in this challenge. Are there some random acts of kindness in there? Things you could do for others? Some way of leaving the world better than you found it? Use the Bucket List 100 to really push yourself well outside your comfort zone and think big.

There's a guy from back in the day called, Henry David Thoreau who once said, 'most men lead lives of quiet desperation and go to the grave with the song still in them.' Don't let this be you. In fact try to remember that life is for living.

The reason for this challenge is to really stretch your mind to the endless possibilities that life has to offer you. It might take you an entire lifetime to complete this exercise. That's fine. You can add things as you go. Just remember to use this list to remind yourself of the life you've lived as well as the one you plan on living.

WHAT'S ON YOUR BUCKET LIST?

Write down 100 things you plan to do with your life. They don't have to be new, you might have already done them. In which case write them down and tick them off.

HOW ARE YOU FEELING?

Circle, tick or cross out

stressed · nervous · tense · anxious · insecure · confused
positive · happy · hopeful · determined · glad · joyful · proud
bored · tired · hurt · angry · irritated · disappointed · annoyed
motivated · eager · excited · content · daring · safe · inspired
frustrated · furious · scared · trapped · worthless · unhappy
calm · grateful · strong · neutral · empathetic · mischievous · alive
regretful · upset · lonely · low · guilty · bitter · shocked · sad
confident · pleased · surprised · relieved · satisfied · energetic

Once you're done, pick one that you're going to do next. If you've not set a goal in entry 1, maybe use this as a starting point.

ENTRY TWENTY-EIGHT
MISSION STATEMENT

There will be times ahead where things will go tits up and you'll question your sanity. But what would you say to you, in the face of a tough situation?

A lot of the thinking behind writing a personal mission statement or manifesto comes from the power of affirmations.

Studies have shown that affirmations change the brain on a cellular level and have a direct link to your health.

Writing your own mission statement gives you a core set of values to adhere to. It's about making a declaration of what you want, what you believe in and what you know to be true about yourself. Remembering all your strengths and what makes you a good person.

Your mission statement should define you as a person and your primary goals in life. It should be a constant reminder of what you have set out to achieve and how you want to live your life. And as time moves on, so can your mission statement. You can update it along the way.

The work you've done in your journal has led to this point. Take your time, write, reflect and edit it as many times as you need. Think about others, the ideal you, your goals, your purpose, your legacy and all the amazing things that make you the man you are.

Write it. Then live it.

WHAT WOULD YOU SAY TO YOU?

Write down what you would say to yourself in the face of a tough situation. Remind yourself of your strengths and positives. Use this next time shit hits the fan.

HOW ARE YOU FEELING?

Circle, tick or cross out

stressed · nervous · tense · anxious · insecure · confused

positive · happy · hopeful · determined · glad · joyful · proud

bored · tired · hurt · angry · irritated · disappointed · annoyed

motivated · eager · excited · content · daring · safe · inspired

frustrated · furious · scared · trapped · worthless · unhappy

calm · grateful · strong · neutral · empathetic · mischievous · alive

regretful · upset · lonely · low · guilty · bitter · shocked · sad

confident · pleased · surprised · relieved · satisfied · energetic

Need some help with this? Head to page 180 to learn more about the power of the Mission Statement.

ENTRY TWENTY-NINE
GAME PLAN

Top teams use game plans to work out how they're going to get the result they want. It's no different for you. You can create your own game plan to win at life.

Be the architect of your own life.

Having a plan has been psychologically proven to free up your mind to get on with other things around you. Once we've mapped out a plan for a specific goal, we can either crack on with it or focus on another goal or another plan or just relax.

Life will just happen with or without you. You can plan for everything and still not have a plan for the events that come along completely off-plan. But at least having some kind of blueprint to work from will give you a reference point. Something to look back at when things just don't feel right, where you can go 'oh yeh, that's what I was planning to do'. And you can pick up from there.

So draw it, map it out, create the game plan that you're going to use to beat the opposition. Top sporting teams don't just go into big games and make it up as they go along. They have highly thought through strategies to win. This doesn't guarantee a victory, but it does give them a better chance of getting a good result on match day.

And it's completely OK to live life without out a plan. If that's your plan — stick to it.

WHAT'S YOUR GAME PLAN?

Where do you want your life to be in 2 years time? Think of what kind of person you want to be, the life you want to live and the things you want to achieve.

HOW ARE YOU FEELING?

Circle, tick or cross out

stressed · nervous · tense · anxious · insecure · confused

positive · happy · hopeful · determined · glad · joyful · proud

bored · tired · hurt · angry · irritated · disappointed · annoyed

motivated · eager · excited · content · daring · safe · inspired

frustrated · furious · scared · trapped · worthless · unhappy

calm · grateful · strong · neutral · empathetic · mischievous · alive

regretful · upset · lonely · low · guilty · bitter · shocked · sad

confident · pleased · surprised · relieved · satisfied · energetic

Drawing a time-line with a start and end date can help. Give yourself realistic dates for the completion of each section too. And then go do it.

ENTRY THIRTY
BACK UP

If this entire journey has proved anything to you, it's that you now have the tools to look after yourself.

No matter what your reasons are for embarking on this journey, you're not alone for any of it.

No matter what you're going through, up or down — there's someone else out there experiencing the exact same thing, at the exact same time you are. And there are people around you that will listen and support you. It might even be the people closest to you, you just don't realise it. All it takes is your courage to kick-off with that first word.

And once these people know where you're at, they'll have your back through thick and thin. Cos' they understand, because they care, because you've fired up something inside of them.

But here's a powerful fact for you: **You've got your own back.**

You've proved to yourself by doing this that you can look after yourself. That no matter what life throws at you, this is your place. A place to look after you.

So if your friends are busy, or you feel no one is listening, or no one could possibly understand what you're going through — there will always be someone that does and that, my friend, is you.

Don't ever forget that.

WHO'S GOT YOUR BACK?

Think about your friends, family and co-workers — do they
support you? Can you talk to them honestly and openly?
How does it feel to know you've got your own back?

HOW ARE YOU FEELING?

Circle, tick or cross out

stressed   nervous   tense   anxious   insecure   confused

positive   happy   hopeful   determined   glad   joyful   proud

bored   tired   hurt   angry   irritated   disappointed   annoyed

motivated   eager   excited   content   daring   safe   inspired

frustrated   furious   scared   trapped   worthless   unhappy

calm   grateful   strong   neutral   empathetic   mischievous   alive

regretful   upset   lonely   low   guilty   bitter   shocked   sad

confident   pleased   surprised   relieved   satisfied   energetic

There's always someone out there going through
the same thing you are. Find them. Talk to them.

FINISH
LINE

If you're genuinely at this point, after completing 30 entries then you, sir, are an incredible human being.

This is no easy thing. I should know, I wrote it and have experienced each of these questions myself. You've been pushed, pulled, ripped out of your comfort zone and had your stamina tested. And I hope you have found this book not just an experience but an actual journey.

An adventure of epic proportions that has led you to find something deep inside you. An inner strength to fight for what you want, for what you believe in, for a version of yourself that you always knew existed. And hopefully this book will continue to guide you.

This is far from over. In fact this is just the beginning. Don't be a stranger to the paper anymore. You can now keep a journal. The rest is up to you. You've got this. Now apply everything you've learned along the way for the rest of your journey.

WHAT HAVE YOU DISCOVERED?

What have you learned about yourself, your life
and the people around you? How have you found
the journey to getting here?

HOW ARE YOU FEELING NOW?

Circle, tick or cross out

stressed nervous tense anxious insecure confused

positive happy hopeful determined glad joyful proud

bored tired hurt angry irritated disappointed annoyed

motivated eager excited content daring safe inspired

frustrated furious scared trapped worthless unhappy

calm grateful strong neutral empathetic mischievous alive

regretful upset lonely low guilty bitter shocked sad

confident pleased surprised relieved satisfied energetic

Have you become a better version of the man you
were at the beginning of this journey?

SUPPORT GUIDE

This part of the book is an additional support guide to help you if you get stuck or feel a bit shit and can't be bothered to write.

It's all cool. I've been there too. Hopefully this will help fire you back up again and remind you that you're OK. My main advice with all this stuff is that you can't get any of it wrong. It's not how well you do something but that you do it at all.

The next few pages will allow you to break away from your sessions, maybe approach your writing or your life slightly differently. It will cover a series of topics that will leave you feeling inspired and reassured.

You'll also find additional support should you find yourself needing to talk to someone. I found that keeping a journal opened up a voice inside me that had lain dormant my entire life. Not talking led me to a point where I imploded into my own black hole where no light could escape. But there was light. There were people around me to help me out. At the back of this book you'll find some people in your area that are there to listen. Use them.

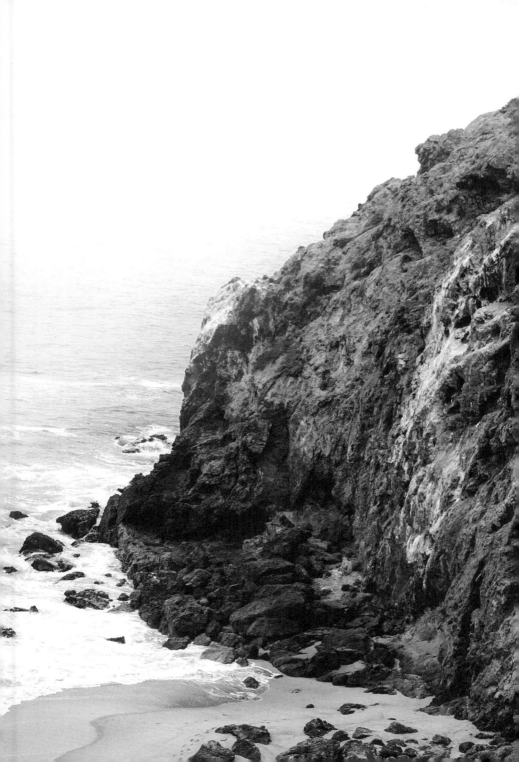

PERMISSIONS

As a kid we associate that our freedom needs to be granted by someone else. We grow up constantly asking for permission to do basic things, like eat food, have fun and go for a piss.

GIVE YOURSELF THE PERMISSION TO DO WHATEVER IT IS YOU WANT.

DON'T WAIT FOR SOMEONE ELSE TO GIVE IT TO YOU.

IT'S NOT THEIR JOB. IT'S YOURS.

We don't need to look for permission anymore though — we're all grown up.

Yet we constantly hold ourselves back. Tell ourselves we can't do things, until someone says it's OK to do so. Think of all the times you've really wanted to do something but didn't. The chances are, either you or someone else didn't give you the permission to do it.

Here's the cold hard fact. It's not the responsibility of others to grant you permission to do things you want to do. You need to learn to give yourself permission to do whatever it is you want.

That could be to feel crap, stay in bed, go sky diving or start your own business. Whatever you want to do you have the permission to do it. You just have to give it to yourself.

This journal is a huge epic adventure. Full of unknowns and endless possibilities. Give yourself the permission to immerse yourself in it, with 100% wholehearted commitment.

It's not selfish. It's necessary.

CHECK YO' SELF

Let's face it, we all check the digital versions of ourselves way more than our real selves. And all this creates is a disconnection from our true selves and those around us.

Try this exercise to check-in with yourself in just a few minutes:

1 Close your eyes and take some deep breaths

2 Ask yourself what feelings you're experiencing

3 Where in your body do you feel these feelings?

4 Acknowledge these feelings and accept them

5 Don't fight them and take another breath

6 Sit for 1 minute and take in your surroundings

7 Breathe and then repeat in a few hours time

To reach your full potential and smash through to your goals you need focus. And the best way to find focus is to check-in with yourself.

Pausing for a moment in your day and asking yourself 'how you're doing' is a great way to check-in with where you're really at. How you're feeling, what you're thinking and how your day is going.

It's an amazing thing to do as often as you can, as it will help you feel grounded and neutralise any negative feelings or anxieties you're experiencing. There's also a boat load of research out there on the positive effects this can have on your productivity and happiness at work.

It's all about connecting with yourself and your surroundings at any given moment — so you're not stuck on autopilot. This exercise is similar to mindfulness meditation. Something I never in a million years thought I could get into. But it's insanely good. Rather than trying to clear your mind, which can sound impossible. You focus your mind on your thoughts and feelings instead. Simple.

I discovered mindfulness meditation via an app called Headspace which uses guided mediation, with the voice of Andy Puddicombe. A normal guy who's been a Buddhist monk, survived testicular cancer and now teaches mindfulness meditation.

My daily check-in exercise and mindfulness time now help when I need some focus. It's also helped with my panic attacks on trains. And all it takes is just a few minutes.

STRESS TEST

It's a known fact that stress is viewed as public enemy number 1 when it comes to our health and happiness.

Try this exercise next time you're feeling stressed out:

Stop what you're doing.

Take in 3 deep breaths from your stomach. In through your nose and out through your mouth.

Then breathe in and out through your nostrils, breathing out longer than you breathe in (count to 4 as you inhale and count to 8 as you exhale).

Whilst in this state tell yourself that the stress you're feeling is a good thing.

But according to some science, it's not stress that's bad for us.

It's actually our personalbelief that stress is harmful to our health — that if you believe stress is bad for you, it will be.

For eight years, leading professors in the US tracked the stress of 30,000 adults. They found that people that experienced a lot of stress had an increased risk of dying by 43%. But only if they believed that stress was harmful to their health. How mental is that!? Talk about mind over matter.

A study by Harvard University found that when you view your stress as a negative, your vessels tighten, reducing blood flow and putting a strain on your heart. But if you view your stress as a performance enhancer, it will help you get through whatever it is you're experiencing, you'll have relaxed blood vessels. Proof that your mind is a massively powerful thing.

So next time you're feeling stressed about something. Try looking at your stress differently. More positively. Tell yourself that stress is good. Stress is your friend and not your enemy.

NEGOTIATING

What you want from your life is not up for negotiation. Don't compromise on it either. It's your life, no one else's.

IF YOU'RE ALWAYS COMPROMISING YOU'RE NEVER GETTING YOUR NEEDS MET.

LEARN THE ART OF NEGOTIATING. AND ALWAYS GET WHAT YOU REALLY NEED.

Compromising is not the same as negotiating.

A compromise is a less desirable option that ticks more boxes, over all the other options that are up for debate. The problem with this, is that no one ever really gets their true needs met. Which sucks. A negotiation is much more clear cut. As you offer something in return for getting what you really want or need.

Setting rules around what for you is non-negotiable is a great place to start. But it's not easy to think of needs that are so important to you that they're never going to be up for negotiation.

Honesty plays a big role in all of this. To be true to yourself and those you're negotiating with, including the people you love.

I've found this a tough concept to wrap my head around. What I've learned through my own journey though is that my health and happiness are more important than other's. For me journaling is a crucial thing I need to do to look after myself. I need the space, privacy and freedom to journal whenever I feel the need to. It's never up for negotiation.

When you're negotiating the needs of others, you're not focusing on your own. It's taken me up until now, writing this book, to realise this. And I'm going to work hard to make sure I stop compromising. To stop letting others hijack my own needs in favour of theirs. And to start focusing on what for me is non-negotiable.

RECHARGE

Sometimes you need to put yourself first. Let people down. If they care about you then they'll understand. It won't be easy. But it will be a hell of a lot easier than continuing on the path to burn out.

Short story

A while back I was properly burnt out from work. A part of me wanted to stop. The other part physically couldn't. It was like a battle with myself. So I took these two versions of myself, gave them names and sat them in a room to have a chat. One was called Plan Man. The other was Field Man. Plan Man is the guy that gets shit done. He believes that without a plan nothing gets done. He doesn't believe in days off. And if there is one, it needs to be planned. Otherwise it's just a waste of time.

Field Man is the opposite guy. He doesn't want to make plans. He's too tired from making plans all day. He's the other side of the same coin. He just wants to stand in a field, on his own and sod all. As soon as I made a plan to do nothing I felt better about doing nothing. I was satisfying those two versions of myself. I'd get Plan Man to ask Field Man what he really wanted to do and Plan Man would make it happen for him.

You need to stop. And it's OK to stop.

You just need to **give yourself permission**. You don't need it from anyone else. Tell your boss. Email the client. Text your friend.

Be honest and explain the real reason why you need to take some time out. The negative response you're convinced you'll get won't be as negative as it is in your head. True story. Once you've stopped, do exactly what you feel like doing. Slob in front of the TV. Sleep. Go for a run. Take the bike out. Listen to music or write. Or do nothing at all. Don't feel guilty about doing nothing. Time wasted is time well spent.

Sometimes though it's dealing with our own expectations of ourselves that prevents us from stopping. Try and think about the parts of you that you make happy versus the parts of you that you don't. Do you constantly 'do' and never stop, when a part of you is screaming for a day off? If so, ask yourself what's the worst thing that could happen if you just did nothing today? Then think about how likely those negative outcomes really are. The chances are they're highly unlikely to actually happen.

By not listening to yourself about what you really want, the only person you're really letting down is yourself.

Now take a day off. Enjoy yourself. Do it — just do it.

PERFORMANCE

Being positive and productive can come with very high expectations. To accomplish the impossible you have to believe that the impossible is not impossible at all. And that requires a lot of energy and positive thinking.

Some people are born with this natural ability to find positives out of negatives. Others work hard at it. But the thing to remember is that it can be learned.

You just have to be mindful of it.

There is a core exercise you can do to give yourself a boost and keep those negative, non-productive thoughts at bay. And they're called affirmations or statements. And they are simple, positive messages you say to yourself.

They reprogramme the negative thoughts and feelings you have into positive ones. It's super simple and could be something you say or write, over and over again. This repetition will help you believe and connect emotionally with your statement.

I regularly say to myself — 'I refuse to not survive. I will not be defeated by life. I will figure it out. There is no other option. I will not stop.'

I don't know where this came from. It's probably a combination of things I've heard through films, music, books etc. But learning to create your own statement or affirmation is a powerful tool to carry around with you on a daily basis. You never know when life wants to try and trip you up and throw dirt in your eye.

Remember to say it regularly. Write it, say it to yourself, yell it out loud when shit hits the fan. Let it give you the strength to get through whatever is thrown at you.

FAQs

When you start something new, you usually have loads of questions – and questions can prevent you from just getting started.

So I thought I'd try answering some common ones so you can stop finding reasons not to write and just get on with starting your journal.

How do I keep my journal private?

Storing it somewhere private such as your sock drawer is always a good start. Unless you want it read, don't leave it lying around. It's a good looking book. But that does mean others might want to look at it. If you're really concerned, keep your journal in a small secure box with a lock on it.

The best way to keep something private though, is by explicitly telling people around you, in your home, what you're doing. Keeping it a secret is never a good idea as it will stir up curiosity and distrust. They will want to know that you're not writing about them. So be honest. Say that sometimes you might be. But that it's a personal and private exercise that you do like meditation. People will respect your honesty and your privacy.

Should I share my journal with anyone, say my partner or family?

Totally up to you man. If you discover something that you feel you want to share then why not share it? Reading it out loud is better than having them read it though. Just in case you don't want them to read some parts of an entry. I often share things I've learned about myself with the people close to me. It's a good way of letting them know where you're at. Use their response as something you put in your journal and think about. Ask yourself, what's the worst thing that could happen if you tell people that care about you how you feel?

How often should I write in my journal?

As often as you feel. Once a day, once a week, once a month. It depends on why you're keeping a journal. Don't feel guilty for not doing it. The more you put pressure on yourself to do something, the less likely you are to want to do it.

For journaling to be effective you have to want to do it. How many times have you gone to the gym or for a run when you didn't really feel like? Sometimes it sorts you out and you find your rhythm but most of the time you just slog through it, with no pleasure, constantly finding excuses to stop.

Don't journal if you find yourself in this mindset. At the minimum, open it up, look at the Thought Trigger and then close it and get back to whatever it is you fancy doing instead. Sometimes that's just as important as writing.

How long should I write for?

Sometimes you'll write for five minutes. Other times it could be an hour. Either way just allow yourself the time. Carve out 15 minutes for each session. If you go over, you go over. You'll feel great for it. And if you finish with time to spare, enjoy the down time you've just earned. Look at the next Thought Trigger and start thinking about it. Time wasted is not wasted time.

Start to learn how to enjoy your own time, in your own company. Don't rush through it because someone is waiting for you. Don't rush through a session full stop. This is your time, you've earned it, now own it.

Some of the Thought Triggers don't apply to me ...

That's fair enough. I've tried to make them as open as possible no matter where you're at in life or what kind of person you are. The incredible thing about MindJournal though, is that people have found how over time their attitude towards certain Thought Triggers changes. One day you might not feel like it speaks to you, but another time it might. Try asking yourself why you can't answer it and write that down. You can always come back to it later.

I forgot to add the date to my entry. Does this matter?

It's a good idea to add it when you remember and make sure to add it before you start each entry. That way you can track your progress over time.

Do I have to work through the journal in the order you've designed?

MindJournal has been carefully designed and structured to build up your confidence in keeping a journal as you work through it, entry by entry. But there are no right or wrongs here. Do it however you want to do it. I won't be offended. You can just keep answering the same Thought Trigger over and over again. Or work through it backwards. Or even upside down. Try it the usual way for the first few and see how you get on.

Everyone has their own way of doing this.

LIFELINES

If you feel you need additional support, that's totally OK. We've all been there. Don't give up on yourself just yet.

You're stronger than you realise.

Whatever you're going through, you're not alone. Help is available and it's OK to put your hand up and ask for it.

It doesn't make you weak, or less of a man.

Australia: Lifeline

Lifeline is a national charity providing all Australians experiencing a personal crisis with access to 24 hour crisis support.

www.lifeline.org.au

Canada: Crisis Line

The professionally trained Crisis Line Responders are there to answer your call 24 hours a day, seven days a week.

www.crisisline.ca

United Kingdom: Calm Zone

This helpline is for men who are down or have hit a wall for any reason, who need to talk or find information and support.

www.thecalmzone.net

USA: NAMI

NAMI is America's largest mental health organisation, dedicated to helping millions of Americans affected by mental illness.

www.nami.org

LOOK AFTER YOURSELF

I created this book for so many reasons. Some more selfish than others. But doing this book has taught me that doing things for the good of yourself is OK.

In life you have to put the oxygen mask on yourself first and then attend to those around you. You have to put your own needs before the needs of others.

I created MindJournal with the intention of helping guys to get writing. Yet along the way I neglected my own needs. I found myself saying yes to things that didn't make me happy. And I wasn't looking after myself. I was so busy making sure that everyone else had their oxygen masks strapped to their faces, I forgot my own.

And guess what got me back on track again?

This very book.

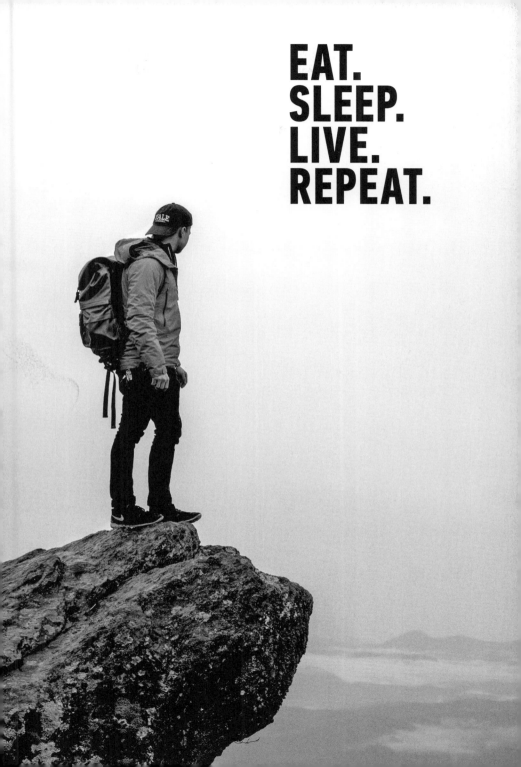

YOU'VE USED ALL THE PAPER

But this isn't the end. This is just the beginning. You've proved to yourself that you can keep a journal. Now keep it up.

Need more paper? Just visit the store
www.mindjournals.com

1 3 5 7 9 10 8 6 4 2

Ebury Press, an imprint of Ebury Publishing,

20 Vauxhall Bridge Road,

London, SW1V 2SA

Ebury Press is part of the Penguin Random House group of companies whose addresses can be found at global.penguinrandomhouse.com

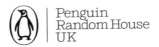

Penguin
Random House
UK

First published by Ebury Press in 2017

www.penguin.co.uk

A CIP catalogue record for this book is available from the British Library

ISBN: 9781785036606

Printed and bound in China by Toppan Leefung

Penguin Random House is committed to a sustainable future for our business, our readers and our planet. This book is made from Forest Stewardship Council® certified paper.

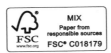

MIX
Paper from
responsible sources
FSC® C018179